Fitness for Busy People

Mema Manna

ISBN:1456593781
ISBN-13:9781456593780

DEDICATION

To my boys....Pino,Mimmo and Sandy.

Your love and support means the world to me

Love you guys....

Table of Contents

ACKNOWLEDGMENTS

1 Brad J. King & Dr. Michael A. Schmidt. Bio Age – Ten Steps to a Younger You.
 Macmillan, Canada.2001.
2 Denise Austin (with Jerome Agel as producer). Denise Austin's 1-Minute
Exercises. Vintage Books/Random House. New York. 1987.
3 Dr. Lynn Goldberg and Dr. Diane Elliot. The Healing Power of Exercise.
John Wiley & Sons. New York. 2000.
4 Goldberg and Elliot.
5 Newspaper article. "The Cutting-the-Fat Issue that Politicians Ignore."
Montreal Gazette. Dec. 12, 2005.
6 Suzanne Schlosberg. The Ultimate Workout Guide for the Road. Houghton Mifflin Co. Boston, USA. 2002.
7 www.brightlife.com
8 Joe Decker. The World's Fittest You. Penguin Group. USA. 2004.
9 Alisa Bauman, Sari Harrar and the editors of Prevention Health Books. Fat to Trim at any Age. Rodale Press. USA. 1998.
10 Denise Austin.
11 www.pmtionline.com
12 www.pmtionline.com
13 www.target.com
14 Joe Decker.
15 Suzanne Schlosberg
16 Suzanne Schlosberg.

INTRODUCTION

Fit exercise into your busy schedule? That's as
absurd as saying that
there are eight days in a week!

First, you've never exercised before or engaged
regularly in a sport;
Second, you've never been into the fitness
crowd and have had meagre
time for such pursuits, and third, you're far too
busy to even think of
exercise.

In other words, **YOU'RE JUST NOT INTO IT**.

Of course your friends talk about it and rave
about the latest fitness
craze, but you've seen it too often: some of them
are on the "on-again
off-again" treadmill / stair master mania, and
you wonder why they
haven't shed the fat that they're desperately still
trying to hide.

Seeing what your friends go through and not
seeing any results, you

cling to the notion that your total lack of interest
is justified.

> You're not the least bit inclined to engage in
> these circus-like contortions
> or do those mindless freestyle strokes in the
> water.
> That would only encroach into your already
> busy schedule of juggling family,
> home and career.
> These three combined –
> husband/children/work are your exercise.

> Yup, we've got a problem.

That mindset is like a seething volcano that's about to erupt. If you stubbornly cling to the notion that the "fat to trim" concept is merely a myth and a figment of the imagination of a handful of oddballs, your health could be going into "eruption mode" soon, like a restless volcano.

Have you looked at your body lately? Have you taken stock of your overall physical well-being? Before tackling the idea of fitting exercise into your busy schedule, it might be better if we start with the concepts of self-assessment and then familiarize ourselves with the disease-prevention aspect of exercise.

Once you've accepted the fact that your body needs overhauling, and that exercise is good for your health – then we can talk about some of the ways that you can include exercise into your roller-coaster existence.

This book in your hands right now (or on your screen!) is your **KEY** to fitting exercise into your life.

And rest assured, this book already assumes that you're a busy person with a life to lead; and that's why the tips in here are **specifically designed to fit in with your busy lifestyle!**

To keep things organized and simple, this book is broken down into five easy sections

Chapter 1

Assessing Physical Damage and   Accepting the Importance of Exercise

Do you think of your body the way you think of your car?

 When a few lucky individuals acquire a sports car that boasts of the best automotive engineering available today, watch them read the maintenance manuals religiously.

They take their car for inspection even if it purrs like a kitten and take it for repairs as soon as something does not feel right. And they're very concerned.

That car is their most prized possession, a symbol of all the long and hard hours they put on the job so they could finally acquire it.

 It cost an arm and a leg, so taking care of it is logically, their # 1 priority.

But how important is the *person* that drives that car? Shouldn't that person – shouldn't **you** – be the #1 priority?

Lifespan and Physical Appearance

The average life span of men and women is 80 years, give or take a few years. The painful truth is, a significant number of men and women look and feel 80 before they even make it to the first half of their life!
You spot the tell-tale signs from their physical appearance:

- Sagging dry skin

- Unsightly posture

- Uneven and unsteady walk (they need to drag around)

- those heavy pounds)

- Aching joints

- sporting the "I'm not happy because I look terrible" look

Now, if their appearance is *this* bad, imagine what the inside machinery is like! Most likely, it's even worse:

- clogged vessels

- inefficient heart

- *mounds* of sugar and fat parked in or around vital Organs

Conditions such as diabetes, nervous tension, high
blood pressure and cardiovascular disease that are

silently brewing.

If fitness authorities had it their way, they'd create legislation to make exercise mandatory as soon as a baby leaves the cradle, not during the teenage years when obesity is likely to strike.

But fitness shouldn't be associated with any age limit. You can start at 10 or at 30 – even at 50 and 60 – the idea being that fitness should not be seen as the cure for a condition that's already come about.
As the saying goes, don't wait for illness to strike.

Assessing How Fit You Are

Brad King and Dr. Michael Schmidt in *"Bio Age, Ten Steps to a YoungerYou"* (Macmillan, Canada, 2001) have devised a questionnaire for assessing physical damage to a body as a result of no exercise.

We will borrow some of their guidelines, which we will summarize here:

Start with the question, "**How do I look**?" Do any of these answers apply to you?

- Am I overweight, looking like an apple or pear?

- Do I have a spare tire around my waist?

    - Has my skin become excessively dry, almost paper-thin?

Next, ask: "**How do I feel**?"

        - Do my joints hurt before or after any physical exertion?

    - Am I constantly worried and anxious?

    - Do I feel tired and sluggish most of the time?

- Do I suffer from mood swings?

- Last question, "**How am I doing**?"

• Are simple walking and climbing stairs difficult?

- Do I have problems concentrating?

- Is running impossible for me now?

- Am I unable to sit straight, preferring to slouch or stoop my shoulders?

You've completed your basic assessment.

Note, however, that other exercise or fitness gurus will have their own parameters or indices for assessing your body's overall state and one isn't better than the other.

As long as they include all dimensions of the self – physical, psychological and mental – they are as valid as the next person's assessment charts.

Turning You into a Fitness Buff!

After going through the assessment phase, you're probably experiencing what some people fondly call a "rude awakening".

If you're not mentally prepared to accept exercise, please *don't* force yourself. Just be familiar with its benefits and when you're wholeheartedly disposed towards giving it a crack in the can, proceed slowly.

"Slowly but surely" is the exercise cult's favorite slogan.

Slowly but Surely...

In fact "slowly but surely" was probably what motivated Denise Austin to come up with her popular one-minute exercises (more on this in a later section) She had two types of people in mind when she designed the one-minute movements:

1. Uninitiated

2. People on the go.

It's a *quickie* society we live in; we want everything quick – **especially exercise**! – and many converts would be willing to include it in their routine for the sake of health, if there were a quick way to get in, and certainly a quick way to get out.

Benefits of Exercise

If you make exercise part of your day, Denise Austin believes you'll already experience some noticeable benefits. These include:

- ✓ Waking up in the morning feeling refreshed

- ✓ Walking with a sprightly gait

- ✓ Having energy left at the end of the day

- ✓ Feeling more optimistic about recreation

- ✓ Sleeping more soundly at night

MORE Benefits of Exercise!

The benefits above are general. Let's examine the more specific benefits of exercise on specific parts of the human anatomy, as described by Goldberg and Elliot:

Exercise prevents heart disease!

The average ratio of total cholesterol to HDL cholesterol (good cholesterol) is about 4.5. If this ratio doubles or reaches 7, you double your chances of developing coronary heart disease. You reduce that risk by as much as 50% if your ratio is 3 or lower.

The lowdown on cholesterol: not all cholesterol is bad. You have the good one (HDL-1 and HDL-2), the not so bad one (VLDL) and the harmful one (LDL). To get your ratios, divide the total amount of your cholesterol by your amount of HDL. The lower the ratio you have, the better.3

Exercise prevents osteoporosis!

Ponder the statistics: 28 million Americans have osteoporosis and of this number, 80% are women. Only ¼ of this 80% know they have the condition and only half are being treated. The annual osteoporosis bill to the United States is $14 billion.

Studies have shown that sufficient amounts of calcium and regular exercise build strong bones. While genetics play a major role in developing the risks of osteoporosis, individuals can control some factors that will help prevent the problem.

Peak bone mass is attained in your 20's. Starting an exercise program while still young, even if you live in the fast lane, will help you avoid this bone disease.

Exercise prevents diabetes!

People are still debating how much exercise an individual needs, but for people with type 2 diabetes, exercising three or more times a week improves fitness and blood sugar levels. If you have type 2 diabetes and are overweight, exercise done with the following parameters would be of tremendous benefit:

intensity of 60%-70% maximal heart rate, with

duration of 30 or more minutes, 4-7 days each week.[4]

The above benefits are only a *few* of the many advantages that an exercise/fitness regimen will provide.

There have been hundreds of documented reports that reveal how people's lives have significantly improved and the remarkable transformation that their bodies experience after they made the decision to take ownership of their weight and fat problems.

In fact, Diane Rinehart (former Toronto magazine editor and writer)
wrote in the Montreal Gazette on December 12, 2005:

"What we're hearing about...is waiting times in emergency and operating rooms for ailments such as hip replacements, heart surgery and amputations.

That's a shame because the fact is, if we dealt with obesity, we wouldn't be facing the epidemics of heart disease, stroke, arthritis and diabetes that clog our hospital waiting rooms and OR's."5

Chapter 2

No Matter How Busy You Are, there are Ways You *CAN* Include Exercise

Feeling overwhelmed by the amount of time your friends and colleagues spend in the gym? Turned off by the idea of a tennis game that entails not only the hour-long match but also getting to the tennis club, changing into a tennis outfit and then showering afterwards?

You think, "That's almost 3 hours – three hours I could devote to nurturing my clients and expanding my sales territory!" The bad news is, being penny wise and pound foolish does not work in ANY circumstance, especially where fitness and health are concerned.

Are those three hours worth skipping during a given week when you know that **years** of optimum health can be yours if you had a positive attitude accompanied by reasonable doses of discipline?

A Simple Exercise Program

Instead of *ignoring* exercise altogether, here's a suggestion for integrating it into your busy schedule. Think of exercise like you think of a major task in the office. Break it up into tinier components.

Instead of spending two hours in the gym or in the tennis court like your friends do, ask your trainer to divide your workout program.

Suggestion A

30 minutes four times a week, i.e.: 20 minutes cardio, 10 minutes weights
(1 muscle group, e.g. legs)

Suggestion B

30 minutes three times a week
Mon: 20 minutes cardio + 10 minutes stretching;
Tues: 20 minutes weights (2 muscle groups, e.g. back and abdominals) +10 minutes of cardio.

Wed: 20 minutes cardio + 10 minutes of Weights (two muscle groups, e.g. triceps or chest, biceps or shoulders)

Suggestion C

20 minutes 5 days a week.

Week 1: all cardio

Week 2: weights

Week 3: Cardio on Mon/Wed/Fri

Week 4: Weights on Tues/Thurs

Repeat the entire cycle when you get to month 2.

Frequency and Intensity

Ideally, one should gradually increase the frequency or intensity, or both.
But if you're busy, and definitely can't spare more than 30 minutes a day, then increase your intensity.

This means if your cardio involves the treadmill, take the notch up 1 level (if you started with level 3, go on to level 4 on month 2).

For your weight training, if you started with 5-pound weights, graduate into 7.5 pounds in month 2.
Then on those days when your day is

not filled with meetings, try to stay an extra 5-10 minutes.

Be realistic with your goals, especially when you're just starting.

Increasing frequency and intensity too soon can overwhelm you, making you want to give up.

Variety is the Spice of Life

Another way to integrate exercise into a busy schedule is to vary the fitness routine.

Variety promotes interest in maintaining your workout schedule.

Without variety, boredom sets in, causing you to drop out.

Variety also enables you to accommodate as many different types of exercises from the wide repertory available from personal trainers, books and manuals – and the Internet – and that way you're able to adopt certain movements that you're most comfortable with.

Walk before you Run...

If you're an absolute beginner, a full blown workout which incorporates cardio, weights, and flexibility may scare or discourage you. The idea is to start with small steps.

Do one exercise segment at a time (refer to our suggestions, item 2 above). Besides, very few people can accomplish a two-hour workout more than once or twice a week.

Another way of doing it would be to integrate your favorite sport (swimming, cycling or walking) during the week and say, a particular activity like yoga which doesn't necessitate jumping into the car and making a dash for the washrooms before cardio classes start.

With yoga for example, all you need is a mat and a quiet room in your house for about 20 minutes.

Time Management

If your schedule gets you up and running beginning at 9 in the morning until six in the evening, this day represents 9 hours. There are 24 hours a day and we're not recommending you get up at 2 in the morning to do your exercise.

But have you ever thought that if you get up at 7 to be ready for 9, maybe you can set your alarm clock 45 minutes earlier, using these 45 minutes to engage in a physical activity? If you do this three times a week, that means you get 135 minutes that you can allocate for exercise.

One easy way to do this is to do yoga in the morning (it requires only a mat and comfortable, loose clothing), or turn on the Jane Fonda CD/DVD, or buy a treadmill (the foldable ones) that you can jump into as soon as you wake up.

Another time management tip: not only do busy managers have back-to-back meetings, they also have luncheon and dinner meetings to meet with clients.

Assess each client. Do all of them really need to be wined and dined?
Is an hour long meeting absolutely necessary?
Can't a deal be negotiated on the phone?

See how many meetings you can cancel or shorten. Then fit your fitness program into those slots that have been freed up.

How about this suggestion: instead of going to lunch with clients every day of the week, why don't you schedule lunch meetings for say Monday and Tuesday?

This way you can incorporate a fitness routine for Wednesday, Thursday and Friday from 12:00 to 1:00 pm.

A brisk walk inside or outside the office building, a quick swim in the neighborhood hotel pool, a Pilates course in the recreational centre, lifting dumb bells while on the phone?

Any of these exercises is better than no exercise. Your guiding principle should be to move, move, and move as frequently as you can manage it.

Cubicle Fitness

Just as ergonomic experts are recommending to office workers to take their eyes off their computer screen every hour or so, fitness experts are advocating getting up from your chair and taking a walk and jaunting up and down the stairs.

When you feel the need to take a break, offer to pick up supplies for your colleagues, take the mail downstairs instead of waiting for the trolley, or think of something you could put in your car instead of waiting until 5 pm.
That way, you force yourself to get up from your seat and walk for a few minutes.

If you look into the private offices of some people, you'll see dumb bells,mats and elastic bands – these are clues that they are doing some exercise while on the job – a good and healthy practice to adopt by busy individuals with hectic schedules.

Family Exercises

On the weekends when you join the family in their activities, try to integrate exercise into these activities: if the children are into cycling, join them for bike rides.

Are they off to their swimming lessons or skating lessons?
See if you can sign up in the adults section, or take a walk outside the recreational center while waiting for them.

Chores Burn Calories!

Who says you can't burn calories while doing housework or gardening?
Take a breather from your hectic schedule and devote some down time to tending to your lawn, trimming your rose bushes, scrubbing the kitchen and bathroom floors, etc.

Walk, don't Drive!

And here's another tip that is popular: park your car far away so you can walk to the front gates of the office, to the entrance of the mall, to the doctor's office and to the post office.

Chapter 3

Busy Traveler? You Can Fit Exercise into your Trips!

Hopping in and out of planes is exercise enough, you say. But that's not the kind of exercise that will condition your heart, make your reflexes and joints more fluid, keep the sugar levels or keep you from swinging from one mood to another!

Nor is it the kind of exercise that will make you euphoric after a good cardiovascular session. You need to counteract the effects of jet lag, artificial air in pressurized aircraft cabins and sky fatigue.
Suzanne Schlosberg says,

"Sometimes your travels help you recognize how humdrum your workout routine has become. At home, it's easy to fall into a rut – to use the same weight machines in the same order, week after week, month after month, simply out of habit. But a trip may take the routine out of your routine. You may have no choice but to try new strength exercises or jog in the pool instead of swim laps.

And you might find these new pursuits so enjoyable that you add them to your fitness repertoire at home."6

Common Obstacles

What are some of the reasons why travelers do not incorporate exercise while they're on the road?

- They're stressed or too tired

- They don't feel comfortable about working out in unfamiliar surroundings

- They don't have access to a hotel gym

But if they made just a tiny effort to change this thinking, they'd be on the road to fitness sooner.

Engaging in exercise allows you to get out of that bubble of meetings, seminars and tours.

Walk when on the Road

When traveling, have a pair of good walking shoes (trainers preferably)so that you won't feel so daunted about getting from one side of the airport to another.

Having the right pair of walking shoes will encourage you to walk up the stairs instead of take the escalator, to walk instead of taking the conveyor belt, and to transfer from one concourse to another on foot instead of taking the shuttle service.

You may not know it, but walking these long distances with your luggage in tow serves as a combination/weight lifting exercise!

Fitness while Flying

Once settled comfortably on the plane, make sure you time your stretching and walking periods.
If it's just an hour's flight, walk around the plane once and do your stretching at the back of the plane; if it's a three hour to five hour flight
 (east to west in the North American continent), try to get up from your seat and walk around at least once every hour, doing leg extensions and trunk/neck movements.

If you're crossing the Pacific or Atlantic oceans, those killer flights need not kill you. Increase the frequency of your stretches and walking.

Airlines such as Japan Air Lines show videos of how travelers can incorporate flexibility movements while seated or standing.

Take full advantage of these videos. The exercises may help you ward off fatigue and jet lag.

A note about DVT

In the last five years, there have been reports about flight passengers, especially in economy class, suffering from DVT – deep vein thrombosis.
The link between confining airplane seats and deaths from DVT (formation of deadly blood clots) has been established by the United Nations World Health Organization. It has nothing to do with gender, risk factors or genetics.
 Everyone is at risk in economy class! 7
This should constitute compelling reason to integrate exercise while high in the sky.

To make exercise possible while traveling, schedule your flights so that when you get to your destination, you don't rush through dinner and then go to sleep.

Try to arrive during the late afternoon/early evening, to give you time to shake off the fatigue from the trip, and have at least an hour to do exercises either in your hotel room or in the hotel gym.

Important "to do" things when travelling

- Be fully rested before a trip – have the usual "to pack" items ready well in advance so you're not scampering for them at the last minute, depleting your energy levels.

- Time your sleep correctly – as soon as you board, get the local time of your destination and set your watch accordingly.
  If it's already night time in your destination, wear blindfolds and ask for a pillow and try to catch a few winks.

- Drink plenty of water – wine and cocktails will only dehydrate you further; note that humidity levels inside aircraft is below 10%, so water is your best bet.

If your job requires you to travel at least four times a month, ask your company's travel department to book you in hotels with gyms or a swimming pool.

Make time out of your travel schedule to insert a workout into your grinding schedule.

Here's a friendly suggestion: get up earlier in the morning and before or after breakfast, head over to the gym and do a brisk walk on the treadmill for 10 minutes, or do the rowing machine (great for the core muscles, back problem reliever) for 10 minutes.

This session is just to wake you up from your travel stupor.
See if you can walk to your business appointment instead of taking a cab (that's another 10 minutes).

At night before going to bed, go to the hotel gym again and lift weights for 10 minutes, to complete your workout for the day.
This way you did your cardio and resistance training, two essential components of a fitness program.

Now, tell us, doesn't a 10-20 minute session sound less intimidating than clocking 1.5 hours in the gym

Working out with Friends

Another friendly suggestion: if you're traveling in a group, ask a colleague if he or she would do a game of squash or tennis with you.
The concierge can give you local addresses of sports or recreational centers in the vicinity.

When there's no Gym!

If the hotel gym is crowded or "temporarily closed for maintenance,"you can still exercise – in the comfort of your room.

Here are some exercises that you can perform:

Turn on the TV or sound system and jog in place; or look up the TV guide and see if some old Jane Fonda or Denise Austin shows are on. Get on with the beat

- Jog in place or jump rope (great cardiovascular workout)

- Conduct floor exercises (described below)

Floor exercise 1:

the Cobra (or back extension). Lying on your stomach as though getting ready for push-ups, keep your hands on your side with palms facing down and fingers pointed forward.
With your hands, push to lift your torso off the floor (ensure you're lifting head, shoulders and chest only).

Keep pelvis on the floor and your head looking straight ahead.

Hold and then release. Repeat 3 times. You should feel your spine lengthen.
Joe Decker recommends not just pressing back with your hands, but also pushing your upper body up and forward.

Do not tilt your head back to look at the ceiling (many people make this mistake). This puts a strain on your neck.8

Floor exercise 2:

Crunch (for lower abdominals). The lower abdominals are the weakest muscles in your torso because they are rarely worked,
and they're the first to sag after childbirth and after menopause.

This exercise will help:

Lying flat on your back with your knees bent, cross your arms over your chest. Squeeze your buttocks, tighten your abdomen and push your lower back into the floor.
Hold for 10-20 seconds, breathing normally. Relax, and then release.

Repeat as often as you can, without overworking yourself.9

Floor exercise 3:

Hurdler's Stretch. Bend the knee towards the front, and then tuck your lower leg in toward the opposite thigh. Stretch gently toward the straight leg.
Do not bounce.

This movement is like the ballet movement when an arm goes above the head gracefully, which stretches the sides of the trunk to increase flexibility.10

If you pick up any exercise book, there will be a rich inventory of exercises you can perform while on the go. Pack this in your bag so you can refer to it for correct form and posture.

Yoga

Yoga on the train? Yes! A news report was published in the Montreal Gazette recently saying how many overstressed Germans still hide behind their papers rather than exercise. We're sure Americans and Canadians are no less guilty.

So these commuters are being taught yoga and relaxation techniques on their way to and from work.

Instructors are now in what the German
government calls "wellness trains"
in southern Germany.

This was an initiative taken by Deutsche Bahn –
Germany's state-owned railway.
The organization decided to offer relaxation and
yoga techniques to calm an anxious work force.

Chapter 4

Exercise Equipment "To Go"

If you're busy but want to integrate exercise into your daily routine, carrying the treadmill around would give you a serious back injury.

We're referring to portable tools that you can take with you to the office, keep in the trunk of your car, or pack into your suitcase:

- elastic bands

- light dumb bells

- jump rope

- inflatable Swiss balls (the small ones)

- an exercise video or DVD that you can play in between meetings

  - Yoga mat.

  - Meditation or relaxation music tapes handy.

  - Exercise tubes with handles (to increase muscle strength) and bow tie exerciser (increases upper body strength).

More Portable Exercise Tools!

The choices in other portable exercise tools are impressive:

- **The Ankle Tough Rehab System** is a set of straps made of heavy-duty elastic, and are cut and stitched to make 2 straps that fit over shoes or bare feet. Set comes with 4 different resistance straps for light, medium, strong and tough resistance levels.
Comes also with exercise manual.11

Flex Bars

A portable exercise gadget that is lightweight. The bars improve grip strength and upper body strength, and allow oscillation movements for neuromuscular and balance training.12

Weighted Vest

A gadget to help you add resistance to your workout. Vest is weight-adjustable with each weight packet weighing approximately 0.75 lbs, and its one size fits all feature makes it deal for both men and women.

Steel shot packets conform to the body, and weight adjustments range from 0.75 lbs. to 20 lbs.13

IMPORTANT NOTE: Buyer Beware!

There are some exercise aids that have been specifically marketed to walkers – things like weighted shoes to add resistance while jogging or brisk-walking.

Before you dole out your cash to buy exercise accessories, speak to a fitness trainer or orthopedist first. Some products can be just commercial hype. This article on www.walking.about.com can shed some light on the subject.

If you're going cross-country driving and the trip will take about 12-15 hours, schedule hourly stops so you can perform some stretching exercises, or go for a 15-minute walk in the neighborhood.
Exercising will energize you, diminishing your need for frequent cups of coffee and relieve eye strain.

Hotels

Back to the hotel scene: some nice hotels have spa facilities that you can enjoy while on a business trip. Reward yourself with a facial or a massage **AFTER** a session on the treadmill or 10 laps in the pool.
This is a great way to unwind for the evening, and an added bonus for the individual on the go.

The old saying, "You have to enjoy your exercise, otherwise you'll give up in no time" has never been truer.

Here's a tip. If you can't incorporate a tennis game or a trip to the gym,how about signing up for dance classes (e.g. ballet, jazz, tap, belly dancing). If you've always loved dancing as a child, wouldn't this be a great way to fit exercise into a busy schedule?

If you don't particularly look forward to being with the gym crowd, a dance class will help you stick to the program.

A good motivator – or exercise aid – is to invest in good dance music tapes. Or listen to selected dance tunes on your iPod while traveling, so when you get to your hotel room, you're pumped up and ready to shake that booty!

Using a Pedometer

This is a beeper-sized device that you clip to your waistband. It measures walking and running distance in steps and miles.
Some models are more sophisticated and equipped with measuring features for pace, total exercise time and calories burned.

A pedometer could motivate you to walk during airport or train layovers because you'll know how much ground you've covered and will encourage you to aim for a longer distance on your next trip.
Joe Decker says he tested 6 models for accuracy and 4 out of the 6 were accurate.
He recommends two specifically: Bodytronics Q25 Electronic Pedometer and the Part Ultrak 275 Electronic Calorie Pedometer.14

Always Carry...

Always have the following items with you as you travel:

- comfortable shoes

- padlock

- foldable, light gym bag

- quick dry clothing

Keep these in your suitcase at all times so you don't waste time looking for them and re-packing them. A busy individual like you need not be unencumbered by exercise paraphernalia that you're hunting for just before taking a flight!

Keep a Record!

A workout log would be nice – just to monitor your progress. When you become pleased with yourself, liking yourself for the small efforts you've invested into improving your physical self, you may want to get into a full-fledged workout program with a trainer.

Show him/her your workout log so he knows exactly how fit you are.

Eating Fit!

Let's not forget your fuel! Don't run low on gas; otherwise your body cannot achieve optimum fitness performance.

Nuts, sesame snacks, protein bars, low-fat muffins, a generous helping of dried and fresh fruit, baby carrots, cereal flakes, oatmeal bars should keep you on the go while exercising.

If you're pressed for time to sit down for a proper meal, these portable foods will tide you over, in a healthy and nutritious way.

Chapter 5

Information/Resources for the Hurried and Harried

The One-Minute Exercises Book of Denise Austin contains quick exercises. While quick food is junk food, quick exercise is not junk exercise and therefore must be scoffed at.
If you can afford to squeeze in only five minutes at certain times of the day, this book is a boon.

Not only does it contain one-minute exercises, it takes into account that you'd want to increase your workout duration eventually, so it includes 5-minute and 10-minute exercises.

The book was published more than 10 years ago, but you still see Denise Austin featured on www.msn.com, so she must tap into some of her older exercise programs. Workout programs never get outmoded or go stale.

They're effective today as they were a decade ago. The book is published by Vintage Books (Random House) and theISBN number is 0-394-74633-
3.
Researcher and fitness expert Suzanne Schlosberg, who wrote a fitness

manual for individuals on the go, did a survey of hotels and airports where the busy traveler can do an abbreviated or full blown workout while they're traveling and waiting for their connecting flights.

Here is some information from her work (her book is highly recommended!).

Fitness-Friendly Hotels

Suzanne Schlosberg performed some helpful due diligence to help the busy traveler by providing the names of major hotels with gym facilities(US only). An extract from that list:

• Four Seasons – 95% of their hotels have pools. All of their fitness centers have cardio and weight machines;

• Ritz Carlton – 80% of their hotels have pools

• Sheraton Hotels and Resorts – pool facility in 95% of their hotels

• Westin Hotels and Resorts – all of their hotels have pools.15

Fitness-Friendly Airports

Schlossberg does not stop with hotel lists!

She also provides a list of airports with massage facilities – you must have seen those massage chairs in strategic locations of large, international airports: Here's a sampling:

- Chicago: O'Hare International Airport – *A Massage Inc*, level 6, main terminal west (near post office); open 7:30 am to 9:30 pm
- Boston: Logan International Airport – *A Relaxed Attitude* –terminal B, American Airlines Side, upper level (hours vary);
- Seattle: Seattle-Tacoma International Airport – *Massage Bar Inc* – Concourse C, beyond security checkpoint, Gates N-16 and N-1

- As for fitness centers in airports and near airports, pages 36-38 of Schlosberg's book, *The Ultimate Workout Guide for the Road* (ISBN number 0-618-11592-7) contains a detailed listing of these fitness centers – to help you do your workout on your next airport layover.16

Plus workout programs that Schlosberg labels "The Time to Kill Workout", "The Timesaver Workout", "The Bare-Minimum Workout" all designed for the busybody!

Websites of Interest

Visit the American Council on Exercise web site
– www.acefitness.com
or call their toll free number, 1-800-825-3636.

They provide resources for fitness products and
services and a list of certified trainers.

Also visit: http://does.ors.od.nih.gov/fitness/.
They serve the NIH community (National
Institutes of Health) and offer classes on yoga,
yoga and aerobics.

Lastly, drop by the Mayo Clinic web site:
www.mayoclinic.com. Scroll down the page and
under the sub-heading "Live Well", click on
"fitness."

Chapter6

How Exercising Can Help With Gestational Diabetes

Unless you already have a regular fitness routine, you probably don't want to start one half way through your pregnancy. But the benefits that you will derive as a woman with gestational diabetes who exercises will make the physical activity worth it in the end. Before you begin any new physical activity or routine, discuss with your doctor any guidelines you need to follow or warning signs you should heed.

You do need to be aware and careful about when you eat and take your insulin in relation to any physical exercise. If you wait too long after eating to exercise you will cause your blood sugar to drop dangerously low.

A good rule to follow at any time – exercising or not – is to have a snack with you to raise your blood sugar quickly.

A good snack is something high in sugar that will raise your blood sugar quickly like a juice box or a piece of fruit.

Have a snack with you that is long-acting too such as a granola bar.

You can also purchase glucose tablets for emergencies when you become hypoglycemic.

The best time to exercise is after one of your main meals. If you can fit in a 15-20 minute walk three times a day it would be idea. But if you cannot try and go for a bit of a longer walk at least once per day.

When at work go for a walk after lunch or schedule a family walk every night after dinner. If you already have an established exercise routine it is probably safe for you to do more but a vigorous or leisurely walk is extremely beneficial.

Exercising will help you keep your blood glucose levels under control and increase your energy. Getting in shape through exercise before delivery can help your labor progress smoothly as well.

After a week or two, there will be improvements in the levels of good and bad cholesterol in the body as well as reduction in the current weight of the person.

Exercising is also considered to be the best way because the use of drugs has known to cause side effects when the person takes this.

If the individual does not have time to enroll in a gym, there are otherways to pump those muscles and increase the heart rate. For starters, men and women can go brisk walking early in the morning or before going to work.

Some offices and hospitals encourage people to walk up one or two flights of stairs instead of using the elevator to go up or down a few floors. If the company where one works in has a big parking lot, the individual can try walking a few yards more instead of taking the space near the door.

During any exercise, it is best to drink lots of water. This will prevent the body from dehydration that often leads to exhaustion. Instead of going to the fountain every few minutes, it is best to bring a water bottle.

This will save a lot of time and keeps the person at pace with the group activity or the work being done on the machine.

Someone once said that health is wealth. By exercising, one will be able to lower the bad cholesterol in the body and live longer than those who choose to do nothing but are aware of the dangers of not making some lifestyle changes.

Chapter 8

An Exercise Plan To Lose Weight

Do you have an exercise plan to lose weight? Two excellent choices to consider are the elliptical workout and the treadmill weight loss workout. Let's compare the two kinds of workouts so you will be able to determine which exercise plan to lose weight works best for you.

An elliptical trainer workout has become very popular and actually has a few advantages over a treadmill. It is less strenuous to the knees, joints and lower back so it is very suitable for people with injuries.

It also works all the parts of your body continuously giving you a total body workout. An elliptical trainer workout is great for cardio fitness and you can get a good workout in a short period of time.

A treadmill workout is still a very popular workout today. Many people buy a treadmill so the whole family can use it. A treadmill workout is perfect for beginners because the intensity in the workout is adjustable by walking, jogging or running.

Treadmill weight loss can best be achieved by exercising within your target heart range zone. Here is how to find the right target heart rate for you. First, you need to find out what your heart rate is while exercising after five minutes. To test your heart rate place your thumb on the underside of your wrist to locate your pulse.

 Count the beats for 15 seconds and multiply that number times four. That number is your heart rate.

To calculate your ideal target heart rate, subtract your age from 220.

For successful treadmill weight loss exercise within 70% of your target heart range zone. Both the elliptical trainers and treadmills help you to burn fat and are perfect exercise plans to lose weight. Exercising not only tones your muscles, but actually gives you more energy for your whole day.

You can purchase treadmills and elliptical workout trainers on the Internet as well as fitness stores.

Both machines are very effective for burning fat and losing weight. Just make sure that you buy quality equipment that will last.

If you are looking to burn body fat and take off weight, these two machines can be a great help for your exercise plan to lose weight.

Chapter 9

Burn More Calories In Less Time

When I work with my clients, one of the key elements that I incorporate into all of our workouts is INTENSITY.

In my view, intensity is the most critical aspect of any exercise regime and can mean the difference between someone who reaches their goals and someone who doesn't.

Increasing your workout's intensity will stimulate your body to burn more calories and induce a greater cardiovascular response.
It will also allow you to have a more time efficient workout.

If you are looking to burn fat and become more toned, then increasing your exercise intensity is critical. Many people have the misconception that if you workout at a higher intensity you will no longer be burning fat since you will be in your "cardio zone".

Whereas, if you keep your intensity low for a longer duration you will burn more fat since you will be in your "fat burning zone".

Let me clarify this for you once and for all. By training at a low intensity (<70% max) it is true that you use fat as your predominant source of fuel.

While exercising at a higher intensity (>75% max) your main fuel source is carbohydrate but you will ultimately burn more calories. And since 1 pound of fat is equivalent to 3500 calories, the ultimate goal is to burn as many calories as possible to create a negative energy balance!

One of the best ways to achieve this intensity is through the use of full body compound circuit training (strength training) in conjunction with interval training (on the cardio equipment). The benefit of full body compound training is that since it utilizes more muscle in any given movement you burn more calories. The intensity of the workout also means that each exercise becomes more challenging as your heart rate is sustained at a much higher level.

Here are a couple of benefits to following an exercise program combining circuit training and interval training. Intervals and circuits vastly reduce boredom.

Traditional steady state cardio training and/or weight lifting can become quite boring. Interval training and circuit training offer more variety and excitement to your workouts.

Interval training increases post-exercise energy expenditure (calories burned following exercise) more than steady-state exercise, which means that more fat is burned. After intense exercise, the body needs extra calories as it works to repair muscles, replace energy stores (i.e. carbohydrate) and restore the body to its normal state (e.g. reduce heart rate).

As this can take many hours, you will keep on burning more calories long after the workout is over. In fact, research shows that metabolic rate is higher for several hours following interval training compared to steady state exercise.

Interval training burns more calories. As an example, 30 minutes on an Elliptical machine using a steady state program will burn roughly 292 calories, whereas 30 minutes of intervals will burn approximately 584 calories! Here is a sample workout that will leave you huffing and puffing.

Warm-up +bike, treadmill, elliptical, rower 5-10 min Circuit (45 seconds for each exercise, with 15 seconds rest between exercises) 5-7 min Lunge walks with lateral raises Plank (on stability ball) Squats with medicine ball shoulder press Push-ups Side Bridges Reverse Pull-ups Burpies Interval Training (cardio equipment) 20 sec @ 100% :

40 sec @ 70% x 5 5 min Repeat Circuit and
Interval 3 times Total Workout Time: 45 – 60
min.

If you would like to experience what an intense
workout feels like then please inquire about the
revolutionary Fitter U MP3 personal training
program!

For a fraction of the cost of regular one-on-one
training, this proven MP3 program will ensure
you get to your fitness goals in less time!

Chapter 10

Calorie Counting Done The Right Way = Weight Loss? Absolutely!

You and I know that losing fat and staying in great shape is a difficult task because it is so hard to stay motivated and it is so tempting to cheat, especially when you can hide the cheating. We dieters have all been in a starving situation when dieting and our mind reasons very quickly why that extra piece of pie is not going to hurt us.
We take it, forget about it and then wonder next day why we didn't lose weight.

For most of us dieting is a constant battle between emotion and reason and when hungry, reason is out of the window and emotion just wins. We do not see the immediate effects of our behaviour and therefore our brain is fooled into thinking that everything is all right. On the other hand, let's say you would get very sick when eating more than you need, overeating would stop very quickly.

Getting sick after a little bit of overeating does normally not happen therefore we need to find a different way to show the consequences of our behaviour. We need to show this in a factual manner, an immediate visual display of the results of our cheating. It is not punishment right away, but over time our brain will be conditioned such that taking an extra piece of pie will give negative weight loss results. Then we will start to understand why we don't lose weight and can pinpoint the causes.

What should this visual display look like? First I like charts, they are very easy to understand and can show trends and correlations between variables. In this chart I would like to see over a period of time, the average calories that I take in per day compared with the average calories that I burn per day.

If the chart shows that the intake calories are lower than the burned calories, I will lose weight and vice versa I will gain weight.

Correlate that with a chart that shows your weight or BMI (Body Mass Index) over time and I have the tool that helps me regulate my food consumption versus my daily activities.

If I add my hunger levels before and after the meals, I can fine tune my meal plans and daily activities. In this way I can sustain my dieting for a long time and preferably it will become my way of life.

I have minimized the hunger pain and increase the pleasure of losing weight and feeling more attractive. There is abundance of free online food calorie calculators. These calorie counters just display nutrition facts and are not going to help you lose weight. Nor is a simple calorie calculator that tries to calculate your calories burned solely based on your weight and average activity level. These are simple little gimmicks that are a waste of your time.

Only when you seriously can track and correlate your calorie intake and calories burned over time, depending on your age, weight, gender, height and individual activity intensity levels can you precisely measure your calorie balance. Seeing visually that your weight loss program works is a big motivator to stay on track. Also you can see immediately when you are off track and you can adjust your situation accordingly. Acquiring great health is a complex task.

Interrelating factors like diet, nutritional facts, meal plans, calorie balance, body reading measurements, supplement and medicine intake, exercise routines, daily activity intensity and costs will make it very difficult for you to see the forest for the trees.

Well designed software that keeps track of all of the above factors and can correlate them will make it very easy to manage your health, fitness, weight loss, muscle mass gain or any goal you have set...

Chapter 11

Cardiovascular Training For Excellent Health

Everyone on the planet has to have aerobic exercise. A healthy constitution and quality way of life requires it. It has a lot of perks and will make you perform improved in all areas of your life. So why should you do aerobic exercise?

Aerobic exercise is beneficial to you by developing the lungs to be stronger by boosting levels of oxygen to the body and the heart by helping it to use that oxygen more efficiently. The word aerobic translates to with oxygen, or with air. Exercise that is less intense and longer in duration is aerobic.

With aerobic sessions, an athlete implements the same big muscle area in a steady motion for between fifteen and thirty.
A maximum heart rate of about sixty to eighty % is the goal to maintain. Swimming, cycling, light running, and walking are some examples of aerobic exercises.

These exercises should be able to be done without someone breathing hard. If you cannot carry on a short conversation while working out, you may be moving it up a level by anaerobically exercising.

Muscle groups get extra blood and oxygen from the body during an aerobic exercise session. Halting all of a sudden in the midst of an aerobic session is not a wise move.
This can lead to dizziness and muscular cramping. After a fairly intense work out, a cool off session is usually a wise idea. Moving in place for a few minutes is a good idea if somebody gets too exhausted during a workout session.
Anaerobic exercise is different from aerobic in that it is usually shorter in time span and greater in intensity. With anaerobics the body wears down faster and muscles build more quickly. Football, soccer, skiing, basketball, and weight lifting are sports considered anaerobic exercises. Sprinting or running is another example. Anaerobic exercise will escalate the chances of the body being sore.

Working a certain group of muscles for a specific amount of time to reach your target heart rate is the point of aerobic exercise. This exercises the heart out better and has the body expend more calories.

The aerobic curve is something some people will often hit. This is when you begin working out and elevate your intensity to the max then slow down gradually. Keeping a continuous heart rate is more efficient.

The lungs and heart endure longer and work more efficiently when they are trained. People who perform aerobic exercise on a steady basis will have to exercise longer to achieve their target heart rate as their stamina increases. People that are only beginning will achieve their target heart rate quickly until their body gets adjusted to the exercise.

Aerobic exercise has so many benefits that it is strange to imagine that we often fail to take the time to do it for ourselves. It controls and lowers body fat, expands our whole endurance, gives us more energy, aids our resistance to tiredness, develops our muscles, and increases our lean body mass. It also aids us mentally by lifting mood, lowering anxiety, reducing depression, reducing tension, and making us sleep better at night.
Who can't benefit a bit from all that? These are advantages that people would all use.
An aerobics class might be a good beginning for people who want to reap the rewards of aerobic exercise and aren't sure how to begin.

In an aerobics class, you can do higher or lower intensity exercise. The class instructor should be able to show class members how to do these moves either way. How much you carry your limbs up during the aerobic session is how the intensity is measured. Athletes must perform at the level of intensity pertaining to their level of fitness and the frequency of their exercise sessions.

This type exercise is without a doubt essential for cardiovascular fitness even though it may be a little hard at first. A good body requires regular cardiovascular sessions and is a continuous process. People who have already achieved good cardiovascular condition can keep this by exercising a minimum of three times a week.

Four to five intervals a week should be the intervals of people who are attempting to lose weight and elevate their level of health.

Conclusion

When you started reading this book, chances are you felt that you could *never* incorporate a fitness program into your busy lifestyle.
 Now, however, the chances are quite good that you're confident, enthusiastic, and ready to start becoming fit!

Remember, please, some of the cardinal rules that we've covered here.

Though we won't recap them all – because you can re-read any section of the book that you wish! – Let's just highlight a few of the most important principles that you should bear in mind as you move forward:

• don't do too much at once; start slow, and build a foundation of fitness

• Exercise for *more* than cosmetic appeal; your inner-body needs to be fit, too (especially as you age!)

• plan ahead and stay in hotels that offer you fitness Equipment

- carry essential fitness tools with you as you travel

- Eat healthy and properly so that you don't "hit the wall" as
you become fit!

- Keep a record of your successes (through a journal or log)

- Exercise with friends or other people who share a common fitness interest with you (and make NEW friends in the process!)

- Manage your time effectively so that you can incorporate a fitness program – large or small – into your daily routine.

Now that you've obtained the information you need, the next step is up to you.
Consult the resources recommended in this book, including the websites, and build an exercise program into your life.

What will your rewards be for your efforts? Statistically, you'll:

➢ **look better**

➢ **feel better**

➢ **have a higher quality of life**

And, in case it matters to you..

➢ You'll be the **ENVY** of all of your busy friends and relatives who want to know how someone as busy as **YOU** has become so **FIT!**

GOOD LUCK AND GET MOVING!!!

ABOUT THE AUTHOR

Mema Manna is an author, teacher, mother and grandmother. After retiring from a teaching career she discovered the exciting world of online business and all the opportunities that running an Internet business can bring.

She wrote a number of books related to her teaching while working for "Victoria University of Technology" in Melbourne, Australia.

Her philosophy is that life doesn't stop at retirement; whatever your age, there are opportunities before your eyes all the time; all you have to do is open your eyes and mind to them.

She is, and has been married for 38 plus years, has 2 lovely sons and 1 beautiful granddaughter. Life is wonderful and interesting, never a dull moment that is for sure.

So here begins another journey in her life.